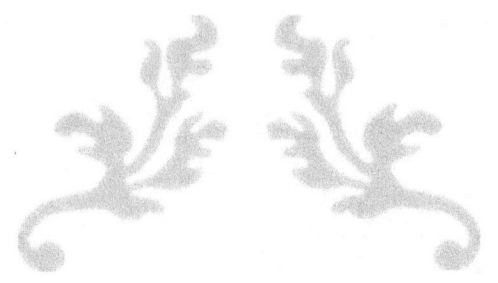

10 LESSONS I LEARNED AFTER
BATTLING WITH CANCER TWICE

Alexander Chase

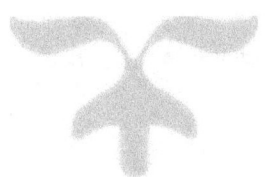

Contents

Introduction

Being diagnosed with cancer can really break you down especially in a case like mine. I have two children that at the time were only 3 and 5 years old, a very difficult situation to explain and quite difficult to understand. I remember waiting in the doctor's room for the report with the results from my last surgery, a report that changed my life and put an end to a very unforgettable experience. People often require a lot of time to process something like this. Some break down in tears while others go into a state of denial and disbelief. However, sooner or later, everyone comes to terms with it.

It is what you do after that realization which is the most important step. I am a survivor, a very proud and happy one, having fought cancer twice before I turned 25 years old. In June 2013 I was diagnosed with cancer. The doctors told me that I had a tumor in the lower abdomen. Thankfully for me, the diagnosis was made on time and the tumor had not grown so much that a simple surgery would do it (as per the doctor). The treatment that followed was pretty straight forward and soon my life returned to normal. However, it wasn't the end of the story for me. Because in March 2014, a scan revealed that I had now a metastasis from the previous cancer, but this time, it targeted the lower lobe of my left lung, measuring about 8 CMs. This revelation really had a massive impact on me. The doctors did not have an answer, it literally felt like the entire world was dropped on my shoulders. But inside I felt that this new cancer was a result of the poor diet, stress, and my overall lifestyle. Thus I had to go through the process all over again but this time a chemotherapy and multiples surgeries were on the way. People who are aware of the effects of chemotherapy would sympathize with me when I say it was the toughest time of my life. But you know what they say, adversity is a great teacher.

Throughout the course of my treatment I had several realizations and epiphanies. I believe that I learned a lot of lessons which enabled me to see life from a different perspective. Because of that I decided to write a short book and share my experiences with you. My aim is not to garner praise or fan following whatsoever. I would just like my story to be heard and if even one of my readers finds the contents useful, I would be overjoyed to know that I have been the instrument of positive change in someone's life.

In the upcoming chapters I will share 10 lessons I learned after battling with Cancer twice by the age of 25.

Lesson 1

Stop Caring About What Others Think About You

One of the most prominent side effects of chemotherapy is that you start to lose your hair. I believe that many of us are aware of the dynamics of cancer treatment but for those who are new to this, I will try to explain. Cancer is caused by damaged cells which start to grow uncontrollably within the body. These cancer cells prevent the body from functioning properly and obstruct the proper functioning of the organ they are affecting. Obviously, the cancer cells need to be destroyed in order to contain this disease and give the patient a fighting chance.

The medications that are used to fight the cancer cells are quite powerful. They have the ability to eliminate the stubborn cancer cells. However, collateral damage is unpreventable. In the process of destroying the affected cells, these medications also annihilate some of the normal cells as well. Usually the cells most affected by the treatments are those which develop rapidly like the root hair cells. So, when you start to undergo chemotherapy, within 2-4 weeks you will start to experience rapid hair loss. And this hair loss is not just limited to your scalp. You can also expect a thinning of the eyebrows and fallout of the eyelashes. Sounds scary, doesn't it? As you can imagine I had to face the scorn of other people, in addition to the physical changes which I was going through.

During the course of my illness, I learned something I should have known all along. People judge you a lot based on your appearance. Seldom would you find someone who would be interested to know what you are beneath the skin. So for most of the passersby, I was an abomination. A hairless man. People seemed to be scared of me and tried to avoid me. I could feel the intensity of their stares, looking at me with contempt as I moved through the streets. At first I really let that get to me. I was finding it pretty hard to cope with the new bodily changes and was not at all ready to face such a reaction from others around me. But then I had an epiphany. A moment of truth that taught me about what I was doing wrong.

So I asked myself, "Why am I letting myself get affected by what others think about me?" And the more I thought about it, the more it made sense to me. I did not owe these people anything. I was not bound to please them or to meet their expectations. Why should I? And this taught me an important lesson in life. You should never let go of your dreams because of what others may think of you.

You may have physical attributes that are distinct from the general public. This does not mean that there is something wrong with you. Instead, it means that you are unique. You are special. You should learn to embrace this individuality. Never let anyone tell you otherwise. There is limitless potential in every human and everyone is born with a special gift. Only by embracing who we truly are can we really achieve success in life.

Lesson 2

Develop An Appreciation For Life

Fighting cancer has taught me some valuable lessons. Perhaps the most important among them all is that I have started to develop an appreciation for life. Our lives nowadays have become so complicated and fast paced. We focus all our energies on work. We stick to a routine that has been forced upon us. Each day we wake up with a ton of worries like how are we going to afford a new car, or what do we need to do in order to get a promotion, etc. And because of this we lose sight of what is actually important in life.

When such a situation arises, we start to get depressed and downhearted about minor setbacks. For example, an office goer might start to feel like a loser if he/she does not have as high paying a job as their peers. Also, kids can easily get depressed if they don't score good grades in their examinations. We as humans have a tendency to become thankless for all that we have and instead focus on all that we have been denied.

My experiences have taught me an important lesson. You need to be thankful for everything that you have been provided in life. Learn to appreciate the beauty around you. Don't be envious of others. In order to supplement what I have just said, I would like to suggest you try a social experiment. I am hopeful that once you engage in this experiment you will start to see things in a different light.

Alright, so what you need to do is to simply take some time off from your busy schedule and go the nearest hospital. Sit in the waiting area, and watch the people come and go. What you will see there will completely change your perspective on life. You will realize that we have all become lost in the cares of the world and have stopped appreciating life. You will see the patients coming in with aches and pains and serious ailments. The doctors look anxiously at their vital signs because any breath they take could be their last. You will also see their parents and relatives, anxiously waiting for word on what is happening to the people they care about. If you would talk to them you would realize that they would give anything in the world in order to save their loved ones from experiencing even a moment of pain. I too had come to this realization when I was being treated for lung cancer. The doctors had to operate and remove the tumor from my lungs. So when I woke up, I found myself full of hoses and tubes. I was dependent on a machine to help me breathe. Now when I reflect back on that time I realize that even this is a blessing that we can breathe on our own. We are independent and do not have to rely on machines in order to live.

How grateful are you for your health? For each breath?

Lesson 3

Be Thankful For What You Have

Man is an envious creature. We are always attracted towards the things we do not have instead of being thankful for all that we are given. Most of us are aware of the phrase "the grass is greener on the other side." Things always look better for our neighbors. This is the reason why we have come to judge people on their materialistic possessions and not on their character.

In today's world success is gauged by your bank balance. The deeper your pockets are, the more you will be respected in society. Gone are the days when people used to value personality traits such as honesty, integrity, and hard work. This can lead to two major problems. Number one, we start to take things for granted and do not appreciate all the good in our life. And number two, we start to lose our identity. Why do I say this, you ask? Well, it is quite simple. When we envy someone and try to imitate them, not in good deeds but the materialistic possessions, we tend to forget our ambitions in life. We forget what things are we passionate about and might end up at a job that we don't necessarily enjoy. You must realize that having money is not everything. You also need mental satisfaction. When you do something, do it with passion and give it your all. That will only be possible when you are interested in that particular task, or when you are doing a job you love.

The second point that we made is that we start to take things for granted. This is especially true for our friends and family. Being busy in the cares of the world, we often don't have time for our family. Parents often have to wait for days before they get a phone call from the children. The small children become desperate to spend some time with their working father/mother. They need positive reaffirmation from their parents and someone who would listen to what they have to say. When someone is diagnosed with a terminal illness, one wish that is common amongst most of the patients is that they want to spend more time with their friends and family.

Therefore we should learn to appreciate the little things in our life. Appreciate your parents, your friends and your children. Spend as much time with them as possible. Remember we came into this world with nothing and we will leave this world with nothing. So our materialistic possessions won't count for anything. Therefore, don't waste your life building up a bank balance that you are not going to enjoy. There are so many ways in which you can utilize money. Go on an exotic vacation with your partner. It might help revitalize your relationship. You might also want to give to charity.

Trust me, there is nothing better to lift your spirits than to see yourself become the reason for someone else's smile.

Lesson 4

Follow Your Dreams

One piece of advice that I would like to give to you at this point is not to live your whole life in fear. If you stop for a moment and reflect back upon your life you will understand where I am coming from. We spend most of our lives in fear. And this is fear of failure and disappointment. Coming back to what we discussed before, we tend to put a lot of emphasis on what others have to say about us. We like to blend in and be one with the society so that we can be accepted.

You need to learn to break free from these chains. Because they stop you from realizing your true potential. For example, maybe you have a great business idea that you would like to try out. But there would be several question marks in front of you. What if you fail? How would you provide for your family without a dependable source of income? And it is these questions that will plant the seed of doubt in your mind. You will start to doubt yourself and your abilities. But I want to tell you that you are better than that. Never be hesitant to take a risk in your life. Because now is the time when you can actually do something. When your life is spent and you are waiting for the end, you will look back and feel sorry for all the opportunities that you missed. So don't let things get to that point. I remember something that I read when I was going through chemotherapy and that is, "Don't wait for the storm to pass. Instead, learn to dance with it."

Going through a traumatic experience also changes you as a person. Maybe before I was not so interested in the problems of other people. However having gone through a life changing experience I can safely say that I have developed compassion towards other people. Especially people who have been diagnosed with cancer. And this is what I would like to advise you as well. Learn to take part of your day to spend some time with those less fortunate than you. Sometimes all they need is someone to share their feelings with. Remember, to smile at someone is also charity.

If you are reading this and you have gone through similar experiences like myself, I would strongly encourage you to come forward with your story. Trust me it is very liberating when you are finally able to open up and share your feelings. Maybe your story will teach someone something that will benefit him/her for the rest of their lives. Or maybe you can be a source of inspiration for someone who has given up.

Lesson 5

Your Body Is Your Temple

You should never take things for granted. I guess this is something that many of you might have had experience with. We are often negligent about the things we have. This also includes our relationships. And as a result of this negligence we tend to forget the importance of the things in our lives. It is only when we are deprived of them that we begin to realize the error of our ways. And most of the times, we realize too late. I would strongly advise you not to make that mistake. But in the context of this book, my main emphasis would be on taking care of your body.

Again coming back to my point, materialistic things don't count for anything if we are not healthy enough to enjoy them. For example, spending all your time at work and not devoting some for yourself is not a good idea. Nowadays people take pride in stretching themselves to the limit. They boast about the all-nighters they pulled and how they are only surviving on coffee and doughnuts. You should not make the same mistake. This is because in our youth, we can often become overconfident about ourselves. However, our body can only tolerate so much.

You might not be aware but having an unhealthy diet can increase the chances of getting cancer. Processed foods and bakery products especially, have been known to cause the most damage. Consuming burgers, shakes, processed meat and microwave products can also disturb the energy balance of the body. You end up eating more calories than what is required. This is the reason why obesity has become one of the most prominent problems in the Western world. Obesity can cause a whole host of problems which includes type 2 diabetes, organ failure, and even cancer. This is why I advise my readers to integrate more fruits and vegetables into their diet.

It is often said that "an ounce of prevention is worth a pound of cure." In light of this, I would like to advise that you analyze the contents of your meals and determine what to include and what not to. Nutritionists strongly recommend the use of fresh vegetables and fruits. These natural foods are loaded with vitamins, minerals, nutrients and anti-oxidants. The anti-oxidants help in cancelling the effects of the free radicals present within the body. The free radicals are byproducts of the chemical reactions taking place inside the body such as digestion, respiration etc. These free radicals can cause disruption inside the body. They can also cause mutations of the cells which then leads to cancer. It is of the utmost importance that these free radicals be dealt with.

Lesson 6

Live In The Present

In order to be truly called healthy, you need to nurture your mind as well as your body. In the previous chapter we talked about how the choice of food can affect our body. In this chapter we will see how developing the right mindset can help. Something which I have learned through the years is that in order to be truly happy, we need to start living in the present.

If you survey the world around you, you will see that mostly there are two kinds of people. There are ones that live in the past. Most of their time is spent wallowing in regret for missed opportunities. They can't help but think about the things they have lost and all the happiness that was denied to them. And because they cannot escape the ghosts of the past, they get stuck. Such people cannot move forward and are plagued by depression and other negative thoughts. And then there are those that live in the future. These people have no care about the consequences of their choices as long as they see a successful future for themselves. These type of people are often negligent about their health and relationships and tend to be more materialistic.

But in actuality, the only people who are truly happy are the ones who live in the present. Now before we move further, I would like to clarify one point. Regarding the discussion above, I did not say that planning for the future is necessarily a bad thing. It is an important prospect of life and you do need to have a plan in order to be successful. However, it is also equally important that you keep things in moderation. Completely ignoring your present self and only striving for the future can have disastrous effects for you. Similarly, not planning at all for the future will also cause you harm. My advice to you here is to remember that balance is the key. You need to plan for your future but that does not mean that you should not live in the present.

There are a lot of things that can help you in this regard. For instance, you should learn to let go of what has transpired before now. Forgive people who hurt you and forget those who left you. Trust me, if you do this you will feel liberated and can definitely move on with your life. Also, remember that in order to achieve your goals, you must work hard. There is no point in making future plans if you are not ready to work for it. Remember, simply worrying about a problem won't solve it. Your rational thinking and shrewd planning will. Try to develop a positive mindset and rebuff the negative thoughts from creeping up inside your mind.

Lesson 7

Take Responsibility

Adversity teaches a person a lot. After going through the fight with cancer, I realized that there was an important lesson for me which I would now like to share with my readers. When you hear the dreaded news that you have been diagnosed with cancer, the human mind can have a temporary breakdown. You might take some time to let it sink in and the bad news might overwhelm you. Your mind will try to find a reason for everything, when there may not be one. You might question fate or God, if you are a religious person. But I believe that this is just to mask some hidden truth.

The point that I am trying to make is that if you have gone through something similar, it is quite likely that you wouldn't have thought that perhaps you yourself played a significant role in the onset of cancer. Now I know this might seem insensitive to you but I urge you to stay with me and let me explain.

Being a cancer survivor, our ambition should be to make changes in our lives so that we can make full use of the second/third chance being given to us. And the only way we can do that is by taking responsibility because a poor lifestyle is the leading cause of cancer. In order to reaffirm this point I will give you my example. I had moved to the United States prior to the diagnosis of cancer. After the relocation, my lifestyle changed completely. And it all seemed so exciting to me. I started to experiment a lot with my diet. I had not realized that I had developed a bit of an eating disorder. I couldn't stop myself from trying all the different kinds of meals available. And as a result, I started to gain weight. Not only that, I had also become so lethargic. I would sit around all day on my couch, watching television and munching down on treats. I also indulged in substance abuse for a while and tried some pills.

Now when we consider all this I think you would all agree that I kind of shot myself in the foot. With such a lifestyle, I think the onus was on me. Yes, you could say that genetics do play a part. But having a poor lifestyle can drastically increase the chances of contracting cancer. Negligence in our daily activities will cause a domino effect. As the detrimental effects start to take hold of your body, your mind will be affected as well. Obese people are often looked down upon by others. This is why overweight people find it difficult to find partners. As a result, they fall down into depression. You would might find it surprising that having a negative mindset can trigger many disorders which eventually lead to cancer.

Lesson 8

Stop Blaming Others

I believe that there are life changing moments in everyone's life. And if we recognize these moments and draw inspiration from them, then we truly will become successful. For me, I think the turning point was when I was diagnosed with cancer. Apart from the usual lessons of life that we learn after going through such an experience, I learned other important lessons as well.

When I reflected back on my life I realized the only thing that was holding me back was myself. I was my own worst enemy. And I think that this is true for most of the people around us. It is very easy to put all the blame on others for your failure. This is because the alternative is quite difficult to accept. It takes a very brave person to accept their mistake. Unfortunately, for most of us, we find all sorts of excuses to mask our failures. Look at the lives of the successful people around us and ask yourself, what do they have which you don't? They too have 24 hours a day just like you. In that time they too have to take time out to sleep, eat and perform other tasks. Hence, lack of time is not an excuse. Similarly if you analyze the other factors from this point of view you will discover that they are nothing more than mere excuses.

So what am I asking from you? It is simple. I want you to take a moment and think about yourself. You need to realize that you have enormous potential and you can achieve great heights in life. The only barrier is your mindset. You need to develop the mindset of the successful people so that you can rise above fear and self-doubt. Once you are able to achieve a positive frame of mind then the sky is the limit.

There are other things as well that can contribute a lot towards your success. Try and discover what you are passionate about. Break free from all the stereotypes. Follow your dreams and be optimistic. You are bound to face some obstacles along the way. Remember, there is no success without struggle. And these obstacles allow you to truly assess how strong you are as a person. Furthermore, you should learn to be patient. Trust me, if you make these small changes in your personality you will definitely feel the difference. Your life will change in a matter of weeks. So do think on this.

Lesson 9

Discover Yourself

Chemotherapy and cancer treatment can take a lot out of you. You lose hair and a lot of weight, in fact, I went down about 40 pounds within the first 3 weeks of treatment. But apart from the physical changes it causes, the treatment can also affect you mentally as well. It is common for cancer patients to have their immune system completely shut down and because of the severity of the drugs, patients would rather sleep most days than face a world that looks down on them for their altered appearance. This reminds me of the time when I was going through something similar.

The treatment had affected me quite severely. All I wanted to do all day was to just lay down in my bed. My body ached and my mind was perpetually tired. I did not have energy to entertain any guests. Nor did I want to share my feelings with any of my friends or family. Those were dark days indeed. But then I read somewhere that "stars cannot shine without darkness" I realized that even at this lowest point in my life, there were things that I could do better.

I convinced myself to not let this phase of my life get to me. Rather I started to enjoy the seclusion. It was a soothing experience. It allowed me the time to reflect back on my life. Now when I write this book, I realize that it was during those days that I really started to get a different perspective of life. I started paying more attention to myself and who I really was as a person. This enabled me to discover my strengths and weaknesses. I started to read a lot. I think this is something that everyone should include in their life. It is better to read books than to waste your time on television watching pointless movies and shows that hardly provide any benefit in the path to your dreams.

Meditation is a great tool to help nurture your mind and body. It allows you to reach a transcendental state when you feel one with your body and soul. I found meditation to be quite therapeutic and if you are going through something similar, I would definitely recommend that you try to meditate at least once a day. Trust me you will be surprised by the positivity. However, if you don't find it effective, there are other avenues that you can explore as well. For example, you can start to write. The topic could be anything as long as it allows you to express your inner feelings. Many of the cancer survivors reading this book will validate my point. Writing about your feelings gives you an outlet to vent out all the toxic feelings and the negativity built up inside you. If you keep a diary, hopefully you will open it up one day and see for yourself how far you have come.

Chapter 10

Summing It All Up

In this chapter, I would just like to sum up all that I have said throughout the course of this book. Dealing with cancer is not an easy thing. I know that firsthand. However, it is important that you learn from the experience and make certain changes in your life. And in order to do that you need to learn to take responsibility for what has transpired in your life. Actions have reactions and you need to make sure that the reactions are not harmful to you or others around you.

We also discussed the importance of having a positive mindset. Humans are not immortals. And everyone who has come this world is going to leave it sooner or later. Therefore, it is important to realize that you should live your life as you want. Do not let anyone dictate to you what you should do or who you should be. Do not be concerned with what others might say about you if you follow your dreams. Never be afraid to make mistakes because our mistakes can teach us a lot and make us better people.

Perhaps the most important lesson that we can derive from all the discussion is that we should learn to become happy with what we have. There is no point in fussing about things that were never meant for you. Spend time with your friends and family and do not become arrogant. In order to stay humble, try to spend time with the less fortunate people of the society. You will start to appreciate the small things in life. Also, try to engage in charity because it can really make you feel good about yourself.

Take responsibility for your actions and be careful about how far you stretch your body. Improve your lifestyle. Eat healthy and take some time out to exercise or meditate at least once a day. The more time and effort you put into yourself, the more you will reap the rewards.

I really appreciate you for taking the time to read my personal experience. I hope that you found this book useful. Remember! Do not lose hope. Stay strong. Stay healthy.